HOW TO MAKE NATURAL SUNSCREEN LOTIONS

DR MIRIAM KINAI

CONTENTS

ACKNOWLEDGMENTS

I would like to express my sincere gratitude to everyone who contributed in one way or another to the development of this publication.

I would especially like to thank http://www.zazzle.com/ChristianArtGifts for their photographs.

1

SUNSCREEN LOTION MAKING EQUIPMENT

Double boiler or water bath

Blender or wire whisk or wooden spoon

Jar with air tight lid

Face mask and gloves

2

SUNSCREEN LOTION RECIPE INGREDIENTS

1 cup or 8 oz or 250 ml water

2 tablespoons or 1 oz or 30 grams grated beeswax

1 tablespoon or ½ oz or 15 grams shea butter

¾ cup or 6 oz or 180 ml vegetable oils with sun protection factor (SPF) like avocado oil, carrot seed oil, grapeseed oil, hemp seed oil, jojoba, macadamia oil, neem oil, olive oil, peanut oil, raspberry seed oil, rice bran oil, sea buckthorn oil, sesame oil, soy bean oil, wheat germ oil and coconut oil

10 ml essential oils with sun protection factor (SPF) like lavender, Roman chamomile, peppermint, helichrysum and myrrh essential oils.

4 tablespoons or 2 oz or 60 grams USP grade zinc oxide powder

*****

3

SUNSCREEN LOTION RECIPE INSTRUCTIONS

1. Put on your face mask and gloves.

2. Heat the vegetable oil, shea butter and grated beeswax in double boiler or water bath until the beeswax melts and mixes completely with the other ingredients. Remove the mixture from the heat and let it cool completely.

3. Put the water in a blender and with the blender on high speed, slowly pour in the cooled vegetable oil and beeswax mixture. Blend until the mixture emulsifies and forms a thick, creamy lotion. If you don't have a blender, you can use a wire whisk or beat the mixture with a wooden spoon until it emulsifies into a thick, smooth lotion.

4. Add your essential oils drop by drop as you blend until you attain your required scent.

5. Add the zinc oxide and stir until it dissolves.

6. Pour your homemade sunscreen lotion into a jar and use as required. Store it in the refrigerator if you want it to last for long. In addition shake your handmade sunscreen periodically prevent it from separating.

*****

4

THERAPEUTIC SUNSCREEN LOTION RECIPES

Normal Adult Skin Sunscreen Lotion Recipe

1 cup or 8 oz or 250 ml water

2 tablespoons or 1 oz or 30 grams grated beeswax

1 tablespoon or ½ oz or 15 grams shea butter (SPF 4-10)

¾ cup or 6 oz or 180 ml vegetable oils with sun protection factor (SPF) like olive oil (SPF 2-8) and red raspberry seed oil (SPF 29-50).

10 ml essential oils with sun protection factor (SPF) like lavender and Roman chamomile essential oils

4 tablespoons or 2 oz or 60 grams zinc oxide powder (SPF 10-15)

Follow the above Sunscreen Lotion Recipe Instructions.

Tips

1. This lotion has a SPF of around 20 though this figure has not been tested and verified.

2. You can also use other vegetable oils with SPF like avocado oil, carrot seed oil, grapeseed oil, hemp seed oil, jojoba, macadamia oil, neem oil, peanut oil, rice bran oil, sea buckthorn oil, sesame oil, soy bean oil, wheat germ oil, coconut oil, hemp oil)

***

Baby Skin Sunscreen Lotion Recipe

1 cup or 8 oz or 250 ml water

2 tablespoons or 1 oz or 30 grams grated beeswax

1 tablespoon or ½ oz or 15 grams shea butter

¾ cup or 6 oz or 180 ml vegetable oils with sun protection factor (SPF) and perfect for the skin of babies like cold pressed organic olive oil and grapeseed oil

10 ml essential oils with sun protection factor (SPF) like Roman chamomile essential oils

4 tablespoons or 2 oz or 60 grams zinc oxide powder

Follow the above Sunscreen Lotion Recipe Instructions.

***

Sensitive Skin Sunscreen Lotion Recipe

1 cup or 8 oz or 250 ml water

2 tablespoons or 1 oz or 30 grams grated beeswax

1 tablespoon or ½ oz or 15 grams shea butter

¾ cup or 6 oz or 180 ml vegetable oils with sun protection factor (SPF) and used for sensitive skin like cold pressed organic olive oil, grapeseed oil and coconut oil

10 ml essential oils with sun protection factor (SPF) like Roman chamomile essential oils

4 tablespoons or 2 oz or 60 grams zinc oxide powder

Follow the above Sunscreen Lotion Recipe Instructions.

***

Dry Skin Sunscreen Lotion Recipe

1 cup or 8 oz or 250 ml water

2 tablespoons or 1 oz or 30 grams grated beeswax

1 tablespoon or ½ oz or 15 grams shea butter

¾ cup or 6 oz or 180 ml vegetable oils with sun protection factor (SPF) and moisturizing properties like olive oil, jojoba, avocado oil, and coconut oil

10 ml essential oils with sun protection factor (SPF) and used to manage dry skin like lavender and Roman chamomile essential oils.

4 tablespoons or 2 oz or 60 grams zinc oxide powder

Follow the above Sunscreen Lotion Recipe Instructions.

***

Mature Skin and Prematurely Aging Skin Sunscreen Lotion Recipe

1 cup or 8 oz or 250 ml water

2 tablespoons or 1 oz or 30 grams grated beeswax

1 tablespoon or ½ oz or 15 grams shea butter

¾ cup or 6 oz or 180 ml vegetable oils with sun protection factor (SPF) and used to manage mature and prematurely aging skin like carrot seed oil and olive oil

10 ml essential oils with sun protection factor (SPF) like lavender and helichrysum essential oils

4 tablespoons or 2 oz or 60 grams zinc oxide powder

Follow the above Sunscreen Lotion Recipe Instructions.

***

Eczema Sunscreen Lotion Recipe

1 cup or 8 oz or 250 ml water

2 tablespoons or 1 oz or 30 grams grated beeswax

1 tablespoon or ½ oz or 15 grams shea butter

¾ cup or 6 oz or 180 ml vegetable oils with sun protection factor (SPF) and used for the management of eczema like coconut oil and jojoba

10 ml essential oils with sun protection factor (SPF) and used for the management of eczema like lavender, helichrysum, myrrh and Roman chamomile essential oils

4 tablespoons or 2 oz or 60 grams zinc oxide powder

Follow the above Sunscreen Lotion Recipe Instructions.

***

Psoriasis Sunscreen Lotion Recipe

1 cup or 8 oz or 250 ml water

2 tablespoons or 1 oz or 30 grams grated beeswax

1 tablespoon or ½ oz or 15 grams shea butter

¾ cup or 6 oz or 180 ml vegetable oils with sun protection factor (SPF) and used for the management of psoriasis like jojoba

10 ml essential oils with sun protection factor (SPF) and used for the management of psoriasis like lavender and Roman chamomile essential oils

4 tablespoons or 2 oz or 60 grams zinc oxide powder

Follow the above Sunscreen Lotion Recipe Instructions.

***

Ringworm Treatment Sunscreen Lotion Recipe

1 cup or 8 oz or 250 ml water

2 tablespoons or 1 oz or 30 grams grated beeswax

1 tablespoon or ½ oz or 15 grams shea butter

¾ cup or 6 oz or 180 ml vegetable oils with sun protection factor (SPF) like olive oil and jojoba

10 ml essential oils with sun protection factor (SPF) like myrrh essential oil

4 tablespoons or 2 oz or 60 grams zinc oxide powder

Follow the above Sunscreen Lotion Recipe Instructions.

***

Menopausal Symptoms Sunscreen Lotion Recipe

1 cup or 8 oz or 250 ml water

2 tablespoons or 1 oz or 30 grams grated beeswax

1 tablespoon or ½ oz or 15 grams shea butter

¾ cup or 6 oz or 180 ml vegetable oils with sun protection factor (SPF) and beneficial for mature skin like olive oil, carrot seed oil and avocado oil

10 ml essential oils with sun protection factor (SPF) and beneficial for mature skin like lavender and Roman chamomile essential oils or beneficial for relieving menopausal symptoms like peppermint essential oil.

4 tablespoons or 2 oz or 60 grams zinc oxide powder

Follow the above Sunscreen Lotion Recipe Instructions.

***

Pre-Menstrual Tension (PMS) and Painful Periods Sunscreen Lotion Recipe

1 cup or 8 oz or 250 ml water

2 tablespoons or 1 oz or 30 grams grated beeswax

1 tablespoon or ½ oz or 15 grams shea butter

¾ cup or 6 oz or 180 ml vegetable oils with sun protection factor (SPF) like olive oil and jojoba

10 ml essential oils with sun protection factor (SPF) and used to manage menstrual symptoms like myrrh, lavender and Roman chamomile essential oils

4 tablespoons or 2 oz or 60 grams zinc oxide powder

Follow the above Sunscreen Lotion Recipe Instructions.

***

Arthritis Sunscreen Lotion Recipe

1 cup or 8 oz or 250 ml water

2 tablespoons or 1 oz or 30 grams grated beeswax

1 tablespoon or ½ oz or 15 grams shea butter

¾ cup or 6 oz or 180 ml vegetable oils with sun protection factor (SPF) and anti-inflammatory properties like hemp seed oil

10 ml essential oils with sun protection factor (SPF) used for the treatment of arthritis like lavender, peppermint, Roman chamomile, and helichrysum essential oils

4 tablespoons or 2 oz or 60 grams zinc oxide powder

Follow the above Sunscreen Lotion Recipe Instructions.

***

Stress Management Sunscreen Lotion Recipe

1 cup or 8 oz or 250 ml water

2 tablespoons or 1 oz or 30 grams grated beeswax

1 tablespoon or ½ oz or 15 grams shea butter

¾ cup or 6 oz or 180 ml vegetable oils with sun protection factor (SPF) like olive oil and jojoba

10 ml essential oils with sun protection factor (SPF) and used to manage stress like lavender and Roman chamomile essential oils

4 tablespoons or 2 oz or 60 grams zinc oxide powder

Follow the above Sunscreen Lotion Recipe Instructions.

Anti-Sadness Sunscreen Lotion Recipe

1 cup or 8 oz or 250 ml water

2 tablespoons or 1 oz or 30 grams grated beeswax

1 tablespoon or ½ oz or 15 grams shea butter

¾ cup or 6 oz or 180 ml vegetable oils with sun protection factor (SPF) like olive oil and jojoba

10 ml essential oils with sun protection factor (SPF) and used to treat depression like lavender and Roman chamomile essential oils

4 tablespoons or 2 oz or 60 grams zinc oxide powder

Follow the above Sunscreen Lotion Recipe Instructions.

***

Mentally Stimulating Sunscreen Lotion Recipe

1 cup or 8 oz or 250 ml water

2 tablespoons or 1 oz or 30 grams grated beeswax

1 tablespoon or ½ oz or 15 grams shea butter

¾ cup or 6 oz or 180 ml vegetable oils with sun protection factor (SPF) like olive oil and jojoba

10 ml essential oils with sun protection factor (SPF) and used to improve mental concentration like peppermint essential oil

4 tablespoons or 2 oz or 60 grams zinc oxide powder

Follow the above Sunscreen Lotion Recipe Instructions.

***

Anti-Insomnia (Sleeplessness) Sunscreen Lotion Recipe

1 cup or 8 oz or 250 ml water

2 tablespoons or 1 oz or 30 grams grated beeswax

1 tablespoon or ½ oz or 15 grams shea butter

¾ cup or 6 oz or 180 ml vegetable oils with sun protection factor (SPF) like olive oil and jojoba

10 ml essential oils with sun protection factor (SPF) and used to treat insomnia like lavender and Roman chamomile essential oils

4 tablespoons or 2 oz or 60 grams zinc oxide powder

Follow the above Sunscreen Lotion Recipe Instructions.

***

Mosquito and Insect Repellant Sunscreen Lotion Recipe

1 cup or 8 oz or 250 ml water

2 tablespoons or 1 oz or 30 grams grated beeswax

1 tablespoon or ½ oz or 15 grams shea butter

¾ cup or 6 oz or 180 ml vegetable oils with sun protection factor (SPF) like olive oil and jojoba

10 ml essential oils with sun protection factor (SPF) and used to repel insects like lavender essential oil

4 tablespoons or 2 oz or 60 grams zinc oxide powder

Follow the above Sunscreen Lotion Recipe Instructions.

*****

5

VEGETABLE OILS WITH NATURAL SUNSCREEN

Choose the vegetable oils you will use for your all natural sunscreen depending on the characteristics of the oil.

AVOCADO OIL

Botanical name: Persea americana

It has a sweet and nutty aroma.

It contains vitamins A, B, D, E, minerals and skin nourishing essential fatty acids.

It has a thick viscosity and it leaves a waxy fatty feel on the skin.

It has an estimated SPF of 4-10

***

Avocado Oil Uses

When used for body massage it is usually used as a 10-25% additive diluted with other carrier oils. It has a thick viscosity and it leaves a waxy fatty feel on the skin.

It is a good moisturizer and is beneficial for normal skin, dry skin, sensitive skin, mature skin, eczema prone skin and psoriasis prone skin.

It is also beneficial for management of eczema.

It also improves the skin's elasticity and is thus beneficial for conditions like solar keratosis.

It nourishes the hair and is especially suitable for use on the hair.

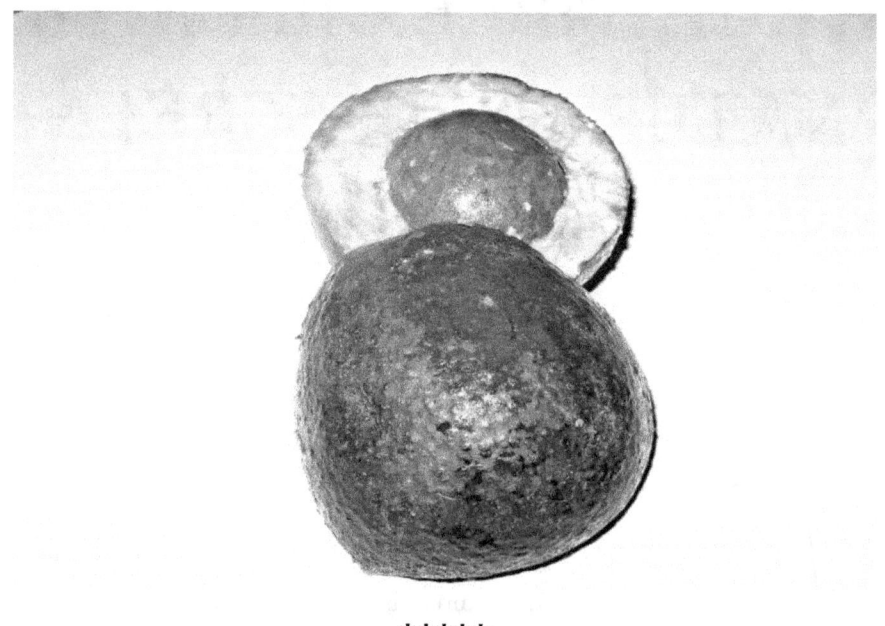

*****

CARROT OIL

Botanical name: Daucus carota

Bright orange in color

It is rich beta carotene (vitamin A) and vitamins like C, D, E with minerals and essential fatty acids

It has an estimated SPF of 30-40

***

Carrot Oil Uses

For massage usually mixed with other carrier oils as a 10% additive

For prematurely aging skin since it is a potent antioxidant with skin rejuvenation properties and it also improves skin tone and elasticity

For eczema and psoriasis since it has anti-inflammatory properties

For burns since it has antiseptic properties, skin rejuvenation properties and it reduces scarring

It also has antifungal properties

It is also useful for itchy dry skin

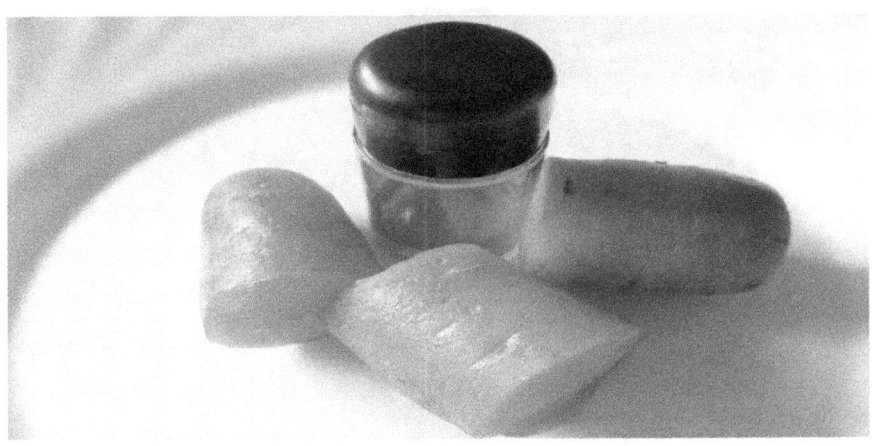

*****

GRAPESEED OIL

Botanical name: Vitis vinifera

Grapeseed oil is made by the process of pressing the seeds of grapes.

It has a SPF of 4.

Grapeseed oil is especially beneficial for oily or acne prone skin.

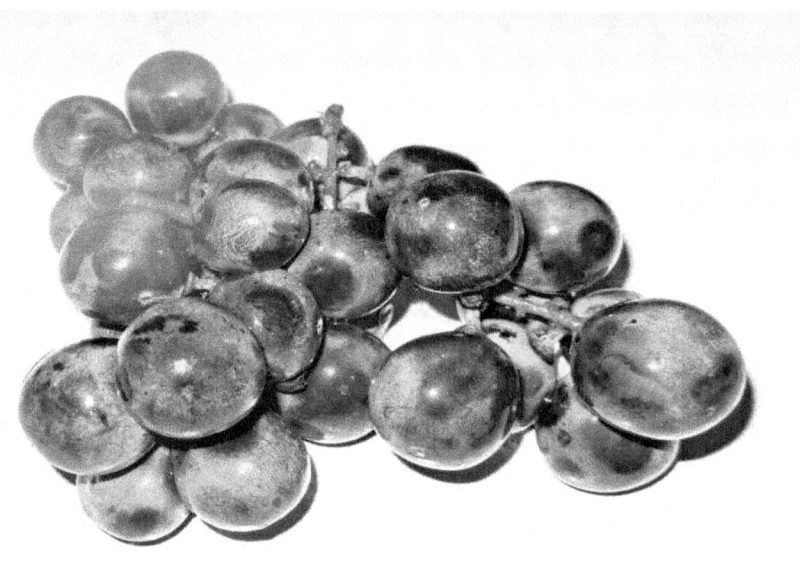

*****

HEMP SEED OIL

It contains skin nourishing fatty acids

It has an estimated SPF of 5-10

*****

JOJOBA

Botanical name: Simmondsia chinensis

It is a liquid plant wax and not a vegetable oil.

Its chemical composition is similar to that of the skin's own sebum or oil.

It has natural sunscreens and a SPF of 4

It has a very long shelf life since it is highly stable, has a waxy nature and antibacterial properties.

It contains vitamin E, proteins, minerals, skin nourishing fatty acids and protective antioxidants.

It has a pleasant aroma.

It is moderately light and has a medium viscosity.

***

Jojoba Uses

For general massage on all skin types and it can be used as a 100% base which means it does not need to be diluted with other carrier oils. It is readily absorbed by the skin resulting in a non-oily softening effect.

It is especially suitable for use on the face and for making face scrubs.

For acne treatment, including back acne, due to its antibacterial properties and also because it is non-comedogenic which means that it will not clog the skin pores and contribute to the development of new acne lesions..

It is also beneficial for dry skin and mature skin.

It also used for conditions with inflamed skin like eczema and psoriasis.

Also useful for excessively oily scalps and hair and scalp conditions like dandruff

It is useful for arthritis due to its component myristic acid which has anti-inflammatory properties.

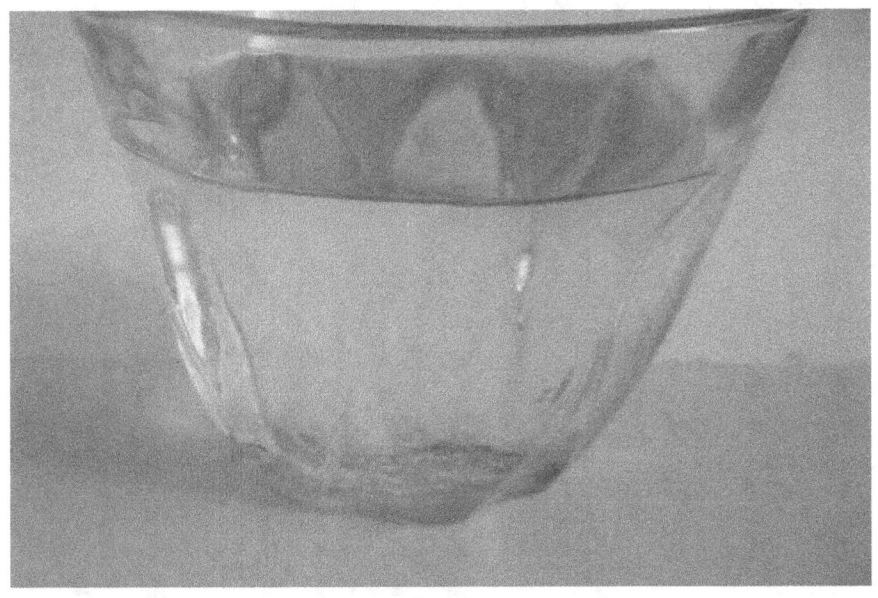

*****

MACADAMIA OIL

It has similar properties to the skin's own sebum.

It has a SPF of 6.

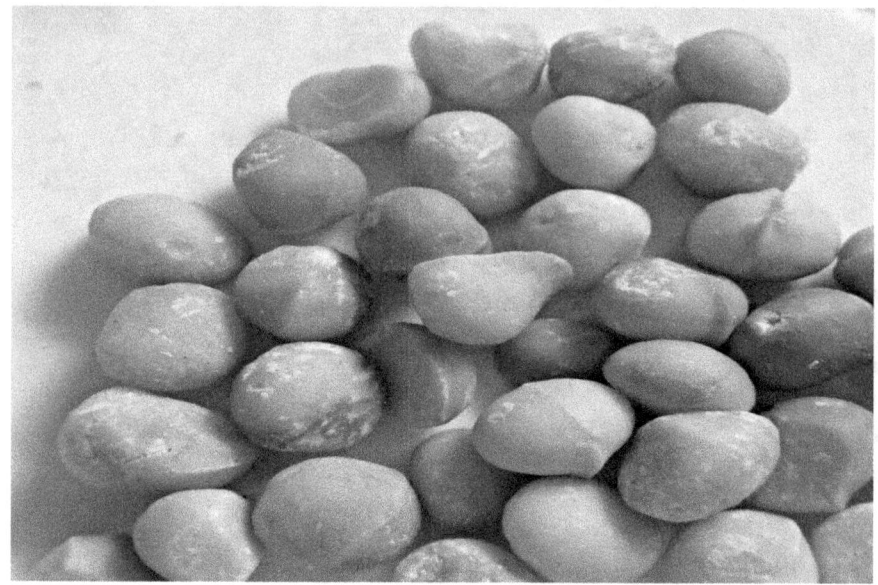

*****

NEEM OIL

Botanical name: Azadirachta indica

Neem oil is made from the seeds of the neem tree.

Neem oil has a SPF of 1-2.

Neem is especially beneficial for oily or acne prone skin.

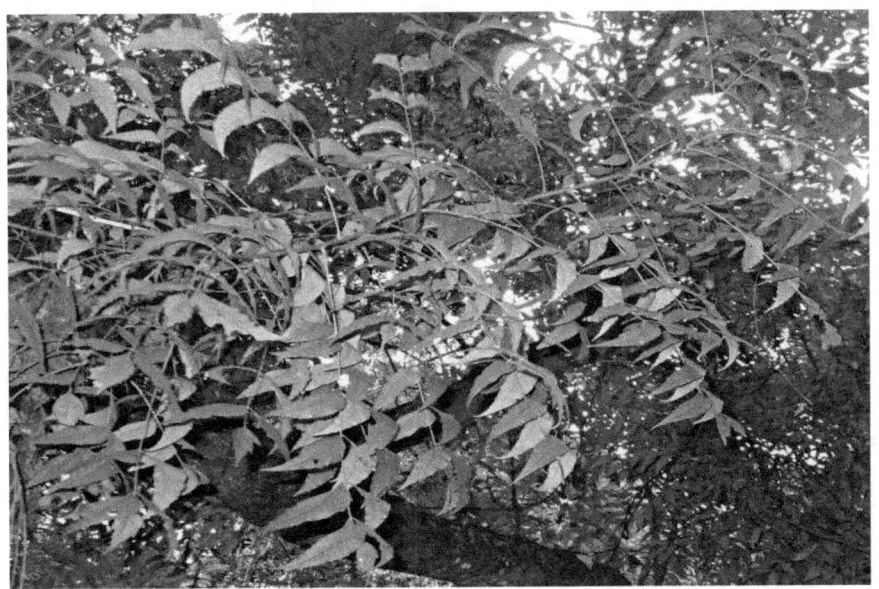

*****

OLIVE OIL

Botanical name: Olea europaea

It has a cooking olive oil aroma.

It has a thick viscosity.

It contains vitamins, skin nourishing essential fatty acids

It has natural sunscreens and a SPF of 2-8

***

Olive Oil Uses

For massage but due to its thick viscosity, it is best used when mixed with other carrier oils as a 10-50% additive.

It softens and moisturizes the skin and is thus suitable for dry and inflamed skin conditions

It is also beneficial for sensitive skin and mature skin.

It is also beneficial for eczema prone skin.

It has been used to prevent stretch marks during pregnancy.

It also softens and moisturizes the scalp and is thus suitable for dry and inflamed scalp conditions. It is also useful for hair conditions as well. It is used to treat dandruff though it may actually worsen it in people with an overgrowth of the yeasts Pityrosporum ovale which feeds on the fatty acids found in olive oil.

It is useful for nail conditions and for making hand scrubs since it conditions nails.

It makes a sensitive soap that it perfect for babies and those with sensitive skin.

It is also used to manage sprains and bruises.

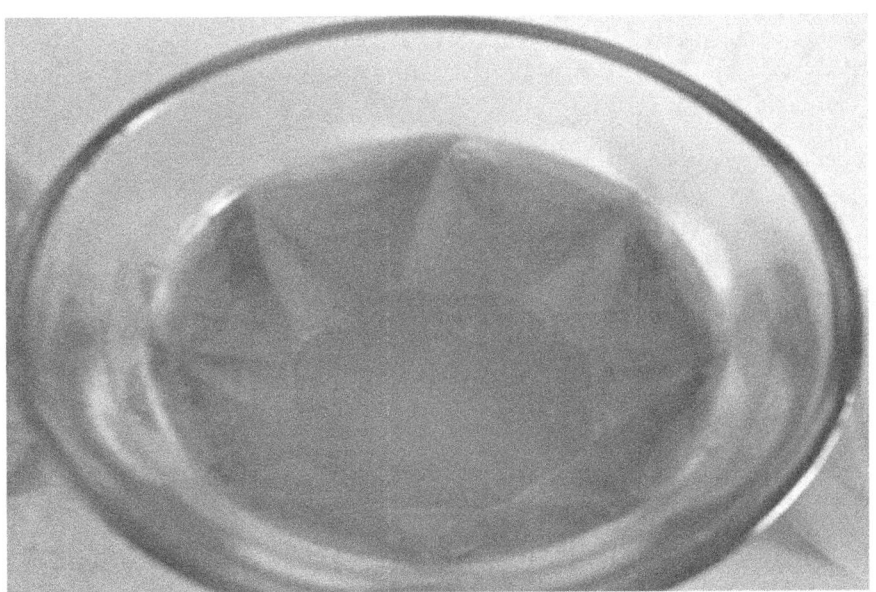

*****

PEANUT OIL

Peanut oil has an estimated SPF of 4-10

*****

RED RASPBERRY SEED OIL

It contains skin nourishing essential fatty acids and protective antioxidants like vitamin E

It has an estimated sun protection factor (SPF) of 29-50

*****

RICE BRAN OIL

Rice bran oil contains a chemical called gamma oryzanol which has a "skin lightening effect" since it inhibits the increase in melanin levels that occurs after exposure to the sun.

It blocks the transmittance of UV rays through the skin.

It has an estimated SPF of 2-10

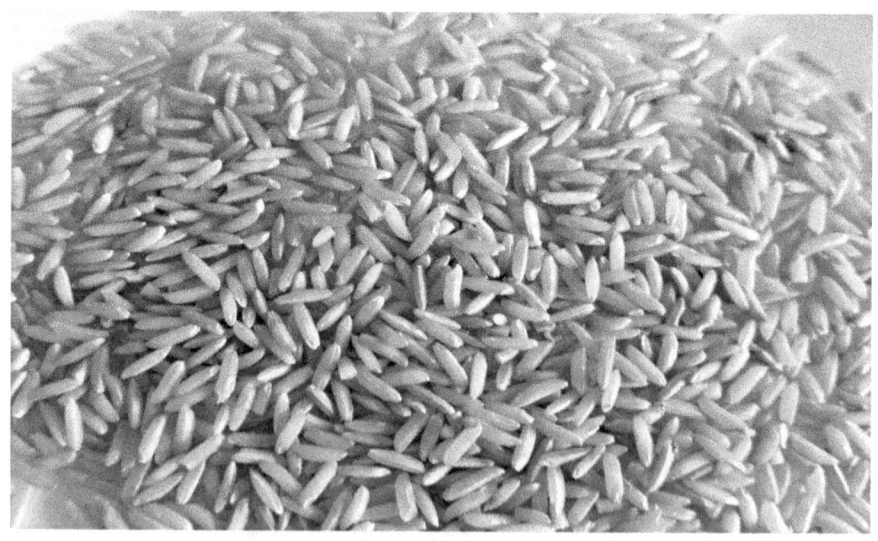

*****

SEA BUCKTHORN OIL

It contains vitamins A, E and essential fatty acids

It has an estimated SPF of 2-10

*****

SESAME SEED OIL

It contains vitamin E

It has an estimated SPF of 4-10

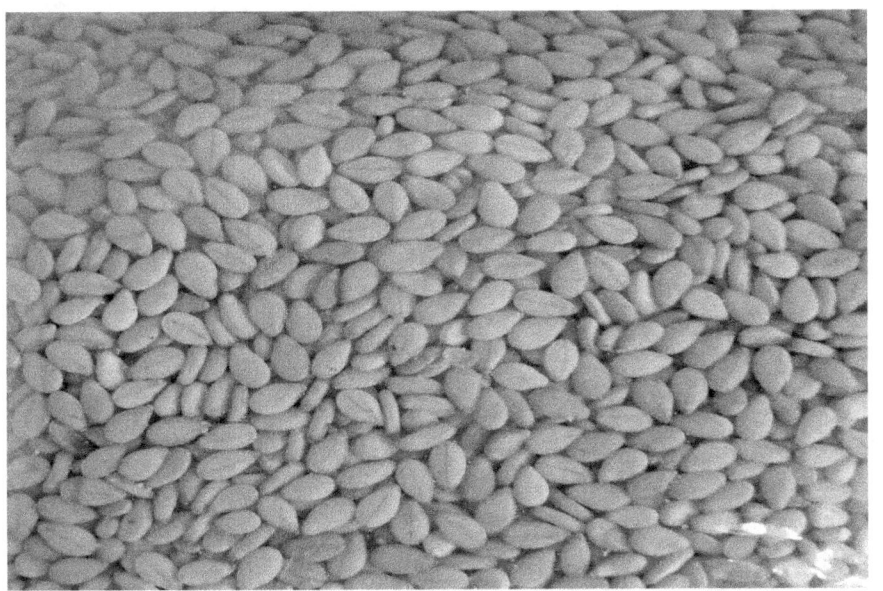

*****

SOY BEAN OIL

Soy bean oil has an estimated SPF of 4-10

*****

VIRGIN COCONUT OIL

Botanical name: Cocos nucifera

It has a fragrant coconut aroma

It is solid at room temperature and melts at 76 degrees.

It contains skin and hair nourishing fatty acids.

It has an estimated SPF of 4-10

***

Virgin Coconut Oil Uses

For massages and it is best used when added to other massage oils as a 10% additive.

For dry skin since it softens and moisturizes the skin.

For mature and prematurely aging skin since it contains anti-oxidants and helps reduce the appearance of fine lines and wrinkles.

For sun protection since it has a SPF of 4 and also to manage sunburns.

For bruises since it has antibacterial and antiviral properties.

For conditions like eczema and psoriasis.

For dry and damaged hair since it conditions the hair. It can be used as a deep conditioning treatment by applying it to the strands and wearing a shower cap overnight. It can also be applied as a pre-shampoo hair treatment for coarse and frizzy hair.

For thinning hair since it is believed to stimulate hair growth by simply applying it to the bald spots three times a day.

For dandruff treatment.

It also conditions the nails and is thus useful for making hand scrubs.

When used for soap making it makes a hard and long lasting soap which lathers well.

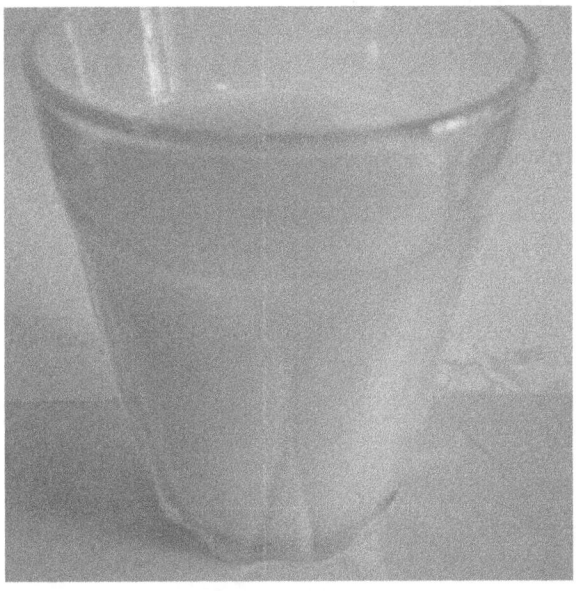

*****

WHEAT GERM OIL

It contains vitamins B, E and K

Its high content of the antioxidant vitamin E protects the skin from free radical damage

It has an estimated SPF of 20

*****

6

ESSENTIAL OILS WITH NATURAL SUNSCREEN

The following are some of the essential oils that contain natural sunscreen:

CHAMOMILE (ROMAN) ESSENTIAL OIL

Botanical Name: Chamaemelum nobile

Method of Extraction: Steam distilled from flowers

Color: Pale green to blue

Perfumery Note: Middle note

Odor Intensity: 9

Strength of Initial Aroma: Medium

Aromatic Description: Sweet, warm, fruity, herbaceous

Characteristics: Nontoxic, non-irritant and non-sensitizing.

***

Roman Chamomile Essential Oil Safety Information

1. Avoid using it in pregnancy.

2. Avoid using it if you are allergic to ragweed.

3. Do not use it alone for more than 2-3 months as it may lead to sensitization.

4. Always buy your essential oils from a reputable vender to ensure you use high quality therapeutic grade essential oils in your blends.

5. Do not confuse essential oils with fragrance oils as the latter are not the natural essences.

***

Therapeutic Uses Of Roman Chamomile Essential Oil

Roman chamomile essential oil has the following health benefits and uses due to its numerous properties:

1. Dry skin type and cracked nipples

2. Skin diseases like eczema, psoriasis as well as inflamed skin from other causes.

3. Surgical scars

4. Arthritis, rheumatism, muscle aches, and neuralgia

5. Premenstrual tension (PMS) and dysmenorrhea or painful periods

6. Menopausal symptoms

7. Stress management to relieve tension headaches and help one relax since its aroma is mentally soothing.

8. Insomnia or sleeplessness

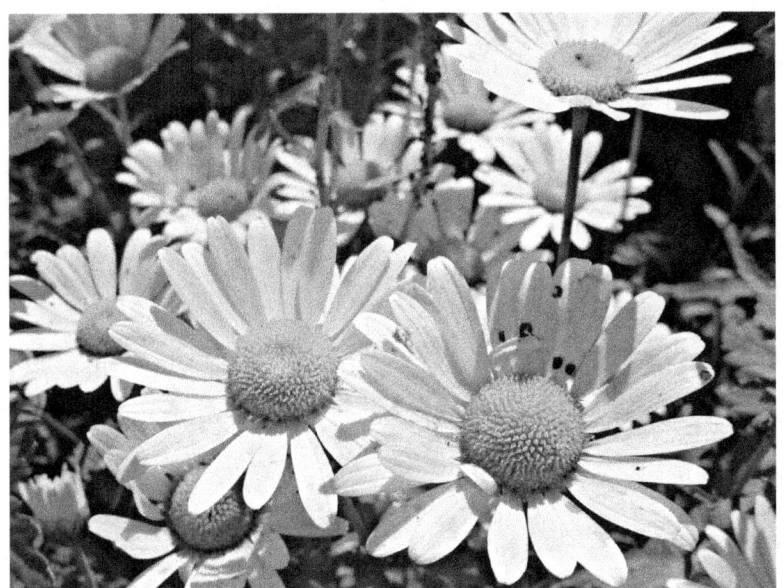

*****

HELICHRYSUM ESSENTIAL OIL

Botanical Name: Helichrysum angustifolium

Method of Extraction: Steam distilled

Color: Pale yellow to red

Perfumery Note: Base note

Odor Intensity:

Strength of Initial Aroma: Medium

Aromatic Description: herbaceous and fruity

Characteristics:

***

Helichrysum Essential Oil Safety Information

1. Do not use it alone for more than 2-3 months as it may lead to sensitization.

2. Always buy your essential oils from a reputable vender to ensure you use high quality therapeutic grade essential oils in your blends.

3. Do not confuse essential oils with fragrance oils as the latter are not the natural essences.

***

Uses Of Helichrysum Essential Oil

Helichrysum essential oil has the following health benefits and uses due to its numerous properties:

1. Skin regenerating properties and is used for cuts and wounds, burns, scars, stretch marks, anti aging products

2. Acne and oily skin management.

3. Boils

4. Anti-inflammatory properties and is used for eczema

5. Analgesic properties and is used for arthritis, rheumatism and muscle aches

6. Expectorant properties and is used for respiratory problems like colds, coughs, flu, bronchitis, asthma

*****

LAVENDER ESSENTIAL OIL

Botanical Name: Lavendula officinalis

Method of Extraction: Steam distilled from the flowers

Color: Clear to yellow

Perfumery Note: Middle note

Odor Intensity: 4

Strength of Initial Aroma: Medium

Aromatic Description: Sweet, soothing, floral and fruity

Characteristics: Nontoxic, non-irritant and non-sensitizing. Can be used on all skin types

***

Lavender Essential Oil Safety Information

1. Do not use it in pregnancy especially the first 3 months.

2. Do not use it if you are breastfeeding.

3. Do not use it on young children as it may cause breast development in boys (gynaecomastia) and girls (pre-pubescent breast development).

4. Avoid it if you have low blood pressure as you may feel drowsy after using it.

5. Do not use it alone for more than 2-3 months as it may lead to sensitization.

6. Always buy your essential oils from a reputable vender to ensure you use high quality therapeutic grade essential oils in your blends.

7. Do not confuse lavender essential oil with lavender fragrance oils as the latter are not the natural healing essences.

***

Therapeutic Uses Of Lavender Essential Oil

Lavender essential oil is one of those aromatherapy oils with numerous therapeutic uses due to its numerous properties. These include but are not limited to:

1. Lavender has mentally calming and nervous tension relieving properties and is therefore useful for stress management, anger management and to relieve anxiety.

2. Lavender has cell regenerating properties which help the skin heal faster and with less scarring and thus it is used for minor bruises, burns, sunburns and cuts.

3. Lavender essential oil has antiseptic properties and thus is used for minor cuts, bruises, burns, insect bites as well as acne and chest infections.

4. Lavender has antifungal properties and thus it is used for athlete's foot and other fungal infections.

5. Lavender has anti-inflammatory properties and thus it is used for eczema and psoriasis.

6. Lavender balances sebum (oil) production and is therefore useful for the management of acne, combination, and dry skin types as well as for dandruff treatment.

7. Lavender promotes hair growth and is used for thinning hair and hair loss conditions.

8. Lavender has antifungal properties and therefore can be used for athlete's foot and other fungal infections.

9. Lavender has an analgesic or pain relieving properties and thus is used for sunburns, arthritis, joint aches, muscle aches, spasms, sprains, backaches and painful periods.

10. Lavender essential oil has antibacterial properties and is therefore used for colds, coughs, and the flu.

11. Sleep inducing properties and thus it is used for insomnia or sleeplessness.

12. Also used to manage depression.

13. Emmenagogue properties or the ability to stimulate blood flow in the pelvic area and thus it is used for premenstrual tension (PMS) and assisting in child birth.

14. Insect repellant properties and thus it is used to repel mosquitoes and other insects as well as get rid of lice.

*****

MYRRH ESSENTIAL OIL

Botanical Name: Commiphora myrrha

Method of Extraction: Steam distilled from the myrrh resin

Color: Yellowish amber

Perfumery Note: Base note

Odor Intensity:

Strength of Initial Aroma: Medium

Aromatic Description: warm, earthy and woody

Characteristics:

***

Myrrh Essential Oil Safety Information

1. Avoid using it during pregnancy since it can act as a uterine stimulant

2. Avoid using high doses since it can be toxic

3. Do not use it alone for more than 2-3 months as it may lead to sensitization.

4. Always buy your essential oils from a reputable vender to ensure you use high quality therapeutic grade essential oils in your blends.

5. Do not confuse essential oils with fragrance oils as the latter are not the natural essences.

***

Uses Of Myrrh Essential Oil

Myrrh essential oil has the following health benefits and uses due to its numerous properties:

1. Accelerates wound healing and is used for chronic wounds, bed sores and ulcers

2. Skin infections like boils

3. Chapped and cracked skin

4. Acne and oily skin management

5. Athlete's foot and ringworms

6. Anti-inflammatory properties and is used for eczema

7. Mouth wash for gum infections, mouth ulcers, toothaches and halitosis

8. Expectorant properties and is used for respiratory problems like colds, coughs, flu, bronchitis

9. Emmenagogue properties (stimulates blood flow in the pelvic area) and is used for amenorrhea (lack of periods)

10. Relieves painful periods (dysmenorrhea) and eases difficult labor in childbirth

11. Hemorrhoids

12. Flatulence, diarrhea, dyspepsia

13. Meditating

14. Christmas room fragrances since the three wise men gave Baby Jesus gold, frankincense and myrrh.

*****

PEPPERMINT ESSENTIAL OIL

Botanical Name: Mentha piperita

Method of Extraction: Steam distilled

Color: Clear to yellowish green

Perfumery Note: Middle note

Odor Intensity: 7

Strength of Initial Aroma: Strong

Aromatic Description: Minty

Characteristics: Non-irritant

***

Peppermint Essential Oil Safety Information

1. Do not use it in pregnancy.

2. Do not use it if you are breastfeeding.

3. Do not use it on children less than 5 years.

4. Do not use it if you have epilepsy.

5. Do not use it if you have irregular heart beats or cardiac fibrillation.

6. Avoid it if you have high blood pressure.

7. Do not use it before using a sun bed or going to hot humid places.

8. Do not store it near homeopathic products as it may affect them.

9. It may cause sleeplessness if used in the night.

10. Do not use on damaged or sensitive skin.

***

Therapeutic Uses Of Peppermint Essential Oil

Peppermint essential oil has the following health benefits and uses due to its numerous properties:

1. Thinning hair and hair loss conditions as it stimulate scalp circulation and stimulates hair growth

2. Colds, coughs, flu, sinusitis and chest infections due to its decongestant and antiseptic properties.

3. Halitosis

4. Arthritis, muscle aches, sprains due to its pain relieving properties.

5. Hot flashes of menopause

6. Nausea and travel sickness since it reduces nausea.

7. Colic, flatulence, indigestion

8. Menstrual cramps

9. Its scent is mentally stimulating and it is used to help relieve mental tension and fatigue and to aid concentration.

10. Depression

*****

7

NATURAL BUTTERS WITH NATURAL SUNSCREEN

SHEA BUTTER

Shea butter is obtained from the nut of the Bulyrospermum parkii tree or African Karite tree.

It has a faint nutty aroma.

It is rich in the antioxidant vitamins A and E as well as essential fatty acids. It also promotes skin regeneration and is used to reduce fine lines around the mouth and eyes.

It contains natural UV absorbers and has an estimated SPF of 4-10

It is an excellent moisturizer that melts at room temperature and is absorbed by the skin easily. It is especially beneficial for dry skin and eczema prone skin.

Shea body butters have also been used for stretch marks, burns and scars.

It supports collagen and thereby reduces wrinkles and other signs of aging and is thus beneficial for mature skin.

It also protects and revitalizes damaged hair.

When used to make soap it creates a hard, long lasting bar of soap with stable lather which moisturizes and conditions the skin. It is used for superfatting soap by adding 1 teaspoon of shea butter to each pound of oils and adjusting the amount of shea butter depending on how moisturizing you want the soap to be.

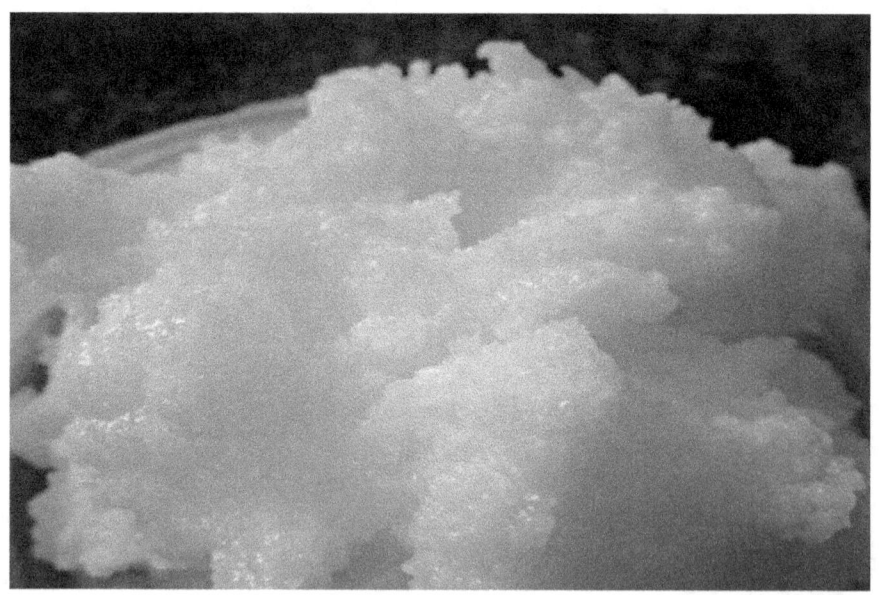

*****

8

HOW TO MAKE NATURAL SUNSCREEN LOTION TIPS

1. Always wear a mask when using zinc oxide so that you do not inhale it since it can cause lung damage.

2. Use vegetable oils with a higher SPF to increase the protection conferred by your lotion. For example red raspberry seed oil has a SPF of around 29-50 while olive oil has a SPF of around 2-8.

3. The more zinc oxide you use, the more sun protection your lotion offers. For example if the concentration of the zinc oxide is 5% the lotion has a SPF of around 5 and a 15% zinc oxide concentration gives the lotion a SPF of around 15%.

ABOUT THE AUTHOR

Dr. Miriam Kinai is a medical doctor and a certified clinical aromatherapy practitioner.

You can visit her blog at http://thetoparomatherapysite.blogspot.com/ or follow her on twitter at http://twitter.com/AlmasiHealth

Email enquiries to almasihealthcare@yahoo.com with BOOKS as your subject.

*****

HOW TO MAKE NATURAL SKIN CARE PRODUCTS VOLUME 1

How To Make Natural Skin Care Products Volume 1 by Dr Miriam Kinai is filled with recipes for making organic bath and body products for normal, sensitive, oily and dry skin types as well as therapeutic products to manage mature skin, prematurely aging skin, cellulite, eczema, psoriasis, ringworms, dandruff, thinning hair, menopausal symptoms, pre-menstrual tension (PMS), painful periods, arthritis, stress, sadness or depression, mental exhaustion and insomnia.

This book also teaches you the best vegetable oils, essential oils, natural butters and herbs to use when making products for different skin types physical conditions. You will learn how to make:

* Bath bombs

* Bath melts

* Bath salts

* Bath teas

* Body butters

* Body lotions

* Body scrubs

* Healing balms and body creams

* Herb infused oils

* Natural soap

How to Make Natural Skin Care Products Volume 1 will leave you with a clear understanding of how to make bath and beauty products to use in your home or to give as gifts or to sell and make money.

*****

THE ESSENTIALS OF AROMATHERAPY ESSENTIAL OILS

The Essentials of Aromatherapy Essential Oils by Dr Miriam Kinai teaches you how to use aromatherapy oils to improve your physical, mental and emotional well being.

The author's experience as a medical doctor and clinical aromatherapy practitioner have enabled her to write a highly informative guide for those who want to utilize the healing benefits of these natural plant essences.

You will discover:

* The safety information and therapeutic uses of 18 essential oils

* How to blend essential oils

* The characteristics and uses of 14 carrier oils

* How to Dilute Essential Oils with Carrier Oils

* How to Use Essential Oils

* Cautionary Measures when using Essential Oils

* Numerous Essential Oil Recipes for bath products as well as skin care and hair care products

The Essentials of Aromatherapy Essential Oils will leave you with a clear understanding of how you can safely use aromatherapy essential oils to heal yourself naturally.

*****

MEDICAL AROMATHERAPY FOR HEALTH PROFESSIONALS

Medical Aromatherapy for Healthcare Professionals by Dr Miriam Kinai teaches you how to use essential oils to treat physical diseases and emotional disorders.

The author's experience as a medical doctor and clinical aromatherapy practitioner have enabled her to write a highly informative guide for those who want to utilize the healing benefits of these natural plant essences.

You will discover how to use essential oils to:

* Treat skin diseases like acne, eczema and psoriasis

* Treat other physical diseases like high blood pressure, arthritis, coughs and colds

* Manage mental and emotional conditions like anxiety, depression, anger and stress

* Relieve the symptoms of menopause and premenstrual tension

* Lessen insomnia and impotence

Medical Aromatherapy for Healthcare Professionals is therefore an essential resource for holistic healthcare practitioners like massage therapists, naturopaths and herbalists.

It is also a useful resource for conventional medicine healthcare providers like physicians and nurses who want to begin practicing integrative medicine and for patients who want to improve their health naturally by using aromatherapy oils.

*****

AROMATHERAPY COURSE

Aromatherapy Course by Dr Miriam Kinai tutors you on how to use essential oils to improve your physical, mental and emotional well being.

The author's experience as a medical doctor and clinical aromatherapy practitioner have enabled her to create a highly informative course on how to use these natural plant essences.

You will learn:

* The safety information and therapeutic uses of essential oils like clary sage, eucalyptus, geranium, grapefruit, lavender, lemon, lemongrass, marjoram, orange (sweet), patchouli, peppermint, Roman chamomile, rose, rosemary, sandalwood, spearmint, tea tree and ylang ylang.

* The safety information and therapeutic uses of carrier oils like apricot kernel oil, avocado oil, borage seed oil, calendula oil, carrot seed oil, castor oil, evening primrose oil, fractionated coconut oil, jojoba, olive oil, rosehip oil, sunflower oil, sweet almond oil and virgin coconut oil.

* How to blend essential oils

* How to dilute essential oils with carrier oils

* How to administer essential oils

* How to make natural healing products from numerous aromatherapy recipes

* How to utilize the healing benefits of essentials oils even if you do not have prior training in aromatherapy

The Aromatherapy Course will leave you with a clear understanding of how you can heal yourself and your family naturally by using essentials oils on your body and in your home.

*****

DARK SKIN DERMATOLOGY COLOR ATLAS

Dark Skin Dermatology Color Atlas is filled with clear explanations and color photos of skin, hair, and nail diseases affecting people with skin of color or Fitzpatrick skin types IV, V, and VI.

Topics covered include Acne Vulgaris, Alopecia Areata, Anal Warts, Angioedema, Aphthous Ulcers, Atopic Dermatitis, Blastomycosis, Blister Beetle Dermatitis or Nairobi Fly Dermatitis, Cellulitis, Chronic Ulcers, Confetti Hypopigmentation, Cutaneous T Cell Lymphoma, Cutaneous Tuberculosis, Dermatitis Artefacta, Erythema Nodosum,

Exfoliative Erythroderma, Gianotti Crosti Syndrome, Hand Dermatitis, Hemangioma, Herpes Zoster, Ichthyosis, Ingrown Toenails, Irritant Contact Dermatitis, Kaposi Sarcoma, Keloids, Keratoderma Blenorrhagica, Klippel Trenaunay Weber Syndrome, Leishmaniasis, Leprosy, Leukonychia, Lichen Nitidus, Lichen Planus,

Lichenoid Drug Eruption, Linear Epidermal Nevus, Linear IgA Dermatosis (LAD), Lipodermatosclerosis, Lymphangioma Circumscriptum, Miliaria, Molluscum Contagiosum, Neurofibromatosis, Nickel Dermatitis, Onychomadesis, Onychomycosis, Palmoplantar Eccrine Hidradenitis, Papular Pruritic Eruption (PPE), Paronychia, Pellagra, Pemphigus Foliaceous,

Pemphigus Vulgaris, Piebaldism, Pityriasis Rosea, Pityriasis Rubra Pilaris, Plantar Hyperkeratosis, Plantar Warts, Poikiloderma, Postinflammatory Hyperpigmentation and Hypopigmentation, Post Topical Steroids Hypopigmentation, Psoriasis, Pyogenic Granuloma or Lobular Capillary Hemangioma, Scabies, Seborrheic Dermatitis, Steven Johnson Syndrome (SJS) and Toxic Epidermal Necrolysis (TEN),

Sunburn, Systemic Sclerosis, Tinea Capitis, Tinea Pedis, Tinea Versicolor, Traction Alopecia, Urticaria, Vasculitis, Vitiligo, and Xanthelasma.

*****

www.ingramcontent.com/pod-product-compliance
Lightning Source LLC
Chambersburg PA
CBHW070612290526
45790CB00002B/884